HEAD PAIN NATURAL RELIEF

Discover WHY You Get Headaches and Migraines
and How to Make Them STOP!

Kathryn Merrow

Copyright 2012 Mind Touch Communications LLC

IMPORTANT LEGAL STUFF

Table of Contents

A brief introduction

It always amazes me that some people never have a headache! They are extremely fortunate.

For the rest of us it's very important to understand HOW bodies work, WHY we get head pain and HOW we can get RID of it naturally.

This book will use the words Head Pain and Headache interchangeably. Migraine is a type of severe headache so sometimes you will see that word, too.

My goal is to make this as easy as possible for you to understand and put into action.

NOTE: If your head pain came on suddenly, is rapidly increasing in intensity, is a type that you have never had before and is very painful, please go to the emergency room right away.

Now, let's start you on the road to getting rid of your head pain and to keep it from coming back and remember:

This is a book for you to use. Highlight parts that apply to you. Fold pages and make notes in the white space. This is your resource to get rid of your headaches and migraines.

About the author

Kathryn Merrow specializes in relieving soft tissue pain. She has provided well over 20,000 therapeutic sessions and utilizes a combination of muscle therapies including Trigger Point Therapy and the St. John Method of Neuromuscular Massage Therapy.

Kathryn isn't a doctor or a physical therapist but she used to suffer as you do and she got rid of her head pain naturally. Having migraines and being a Neuromuscular Massage Therapist gave Kathryn an advantage because she learned how bodies *really* work and which natural treatments work best.

She loves sharing the valuable information she has discovered over the years so that readers can get rid of their pain naturally.

This book is the first in a series of natural self-help pain relief books by Kathryn. You can find her at www.ThePainReliefCoach.com.

What's causing YOUR head pain?

A symptom is something like head pain, numbness or tingling. Symptoms have causes or reasons. Instead of just treating or masking the symptom it's important to figure out the cause of the symptom and get rid of it.

The most obvious cause of your pain may also have a cause. So sometimes you have to look for the cause of the cause.

Here's a list of several possible reasons that your head hurts:

1. Muscle strain. But what causes muscle strain? Poor posture. But what causes poor posture? A weak back or bad habits when sitting and standing. We will talk about that more.

2. Certain foods can cause reactions in blood vessels that lead to headaches.

3. Taking too much headache pain medication can cause rebound headaches.

4. Being constipated. A diet that has too much processed food and not enough fiber can cause constipation. So can too little water, certain medications and poor posture. When your posture collapses it squashes your intestines so stuff cannot move as it should.

5. Aspirin deficiency. Just teasing. There is no such thing as aspirin deficiency even though that's what some aspirin manufacturers may want you to believe. We are not supposed to have 'common everyday headaches'.

6. Losing the natural curves in your lower back and neck. You are supposed to have a little space behind your waist and behind your neck. If you don't, it's often referred to as 'military neck'–too straight. Your neck and lower back reflect each other so if your lower back is too flat your neck curve will also be out of the optimal position.

7. Having too much of a curve in your lower back or neck. There is a fine line between too much and too little curve in your spine. What causes too much or too little curve? Muscles. Habits. Car seats.

8. Sleeping in a way that aggravates your neck muscles, such as curled into a ball with your chin tucked to your chest.

9. Having a leg length difference or scoliosis or tight muscles on one side of your waist.

10. Trigger points in muscles and other soft tissues.

11. Tight muscles in your upper back and neck. If your shoulders feel like rocks, there is a reason and you can fix it!

12. Sitting on a killer couch or car seat.

13. The diet sweetener aspartame. If you are using aspartame please stop right now.

14. Hormones. If you are a woman who has a monthly cycle hormones can play a big part in your head pain. Even so, the more of the other causes you eliminate the less your head pain will be with hormone shifts.

15. High blood pressure. You must see a doctor. Now! This type of headache causes a whole-head, dull, aching, throbbing, tension-type headache feeling. This headache doesn't go away by itself.

16. Hiking your shoulder to hold up your shoulder bag. Carrying too much weight in a backpack with your head sticking out in front to balance the load.

17. Holding the phone between your ear and shoulder.

18. Pressure on nerves can cause head pain. Tight muscles press on nerves. Bones can, too. (Muscles move bones out of place.)

19. Sleeping on your side; always sleeping on the same side.

20. Sleeping on your back with a pillow that is too fat and pushes your head forward and strains your neck muscles; sleeping on your back with no neck support which also can strain neck muscles.

21. Letting your head drift out in front when you exercise.

22. Doing sit-ups and crunches. (But it's okay to do reverse crunches; they won't aggravate your neck.)

We will talk about most of these in more detail (except for #15.)

If you can figure out the cause of your head pain there's a really, really good chance you can get rid of it.

Can you get rid of headaches naturally?

I did and there is a very good chance that you can, too. I used to have horrible headaches. They took days out of my life, three at a time. They don't anymore. But if I do get a headache from a bad position it's much smaller and goes away quickly.

So there IS hope for freedom from bad headaches and migraines!

You have probably heard conventional medical advice. Maybe you have been treated by your doctor for head pain but you still have it. The problem is that conventional medicine usually overlooks the roles of muscles in head pain.

And muscles are responsible for most of our pain.

I cannot see what you look like but here are my best long distance guesses:

Your posture isn't so great. You probably need to correct your posture when standing, walking, sitting, working and sleeping. Tip: If you lift your breastbone and the crown of your head that will help get your head back where it belongs.

And I KNOW it can be hard to correct your posture when you are hurting! It just might not feel possible to straighten up when you have head pain. Your muscles might be pulling you into uncomfortable positions.

But if you can lift your chest and squeeze your shoulder blades together you may feel a sense of immediate relief.

Many muscle therapists (massage therapists) can help release the muscles that are keeping you stuck in poor posture. You can learn to do a lot of it yourself but it requires more dedication and work to do it yourself. But I have faith in you!

Here's what helped my own horrible headaches the most:

1. Extensive bodywork helped straighten me out. I had a side-to-side curvature in my spine (scoliosis) and had about 10 hours of Neuromuscular Massage. (My curve was caused by a leg length difference which was caused by a flat arch in one foot.) The treatment worked deeply into the structural muscles that caused my spinal curves to let them relax and go back to normal resting lengths. This is not comfortable work because your muscles may be very tight but there is such a sense of relaxation after treatment. Your body says, "I needed that!"

2. Elimination of the potential dietary causes: nuts, pork, caffeine (which is in lots of headache medications), chocolate, peanuts, shellfish and some other trigger foods. Sometimes it's easy to see the food tie-in but sometimes it's not. Look for a list of migraine trigger foods online and keep a food diary.

3. Arch supports in my shoes (orthotics) corrected my one flat arch. That, in turn, corrected my leg length difference and that took pressure off my head.

4. My posture was awful. I had rounded shoulders and a forward head. No wonder I had head pain! My muscles were complaining big time! I had to strengthen my back side from my knees to base of the head and relax the muscles in the front of my upper body. Now my head is over my shoulders where it belongs. That takes the strain off the muscles in my upper back and neck and head.

And that means no more migraines!

You will have a similar list which may be shorter or longer than mine.

You see, bodies are really logical. There are reasons you have head pain. When you figure out the reasons and get rid of them, your head pain can be gone.

Migraines in children (and adults, too)

More adults than ever have head pain and I'm sad to say that children are also getting migraines at younger and younger ages. Why?

One of my clients took her 6-year old granddaughter to the pediatrician. The little girl gets migraine headaches that make her sick. This shouldn't happen to a child! It's bad enough when an adult gets a migraine.

What did the doctor say?

He said, "We are seeing more and more children this young with migraines. It's because of all the chemicals in the food now."

That is important!

Here are more possible causes for head pain:

1. Chemicals and other food additives. These are actually designed and produced in chemistry labs for the purposes of either prolonging shelf-life or enhancing the taste of a processed food. If something "tastes good," people will buy more and the chemical companies and food processing manufacturers will make more money. Diet sweeteners are a big cause of migraines in adults; no doubt, also in children with their much smaller bodies.

I must tell you, I'm all in favor of successful businesses and making a profit but NOT at the risk of our health!

2. Magnesium deficiency. All of the vitamins and minerals we USED to get are necessary for our health and wellness. A lot of the things that are sold as food in grocery stores nowadays really aren't food. They are depleted of minerals and nutrients so we don't get nutrients we need unless we eat real food. What's real? Vegetables, fruits, things that grew rather than came from factories. Magnesium is a mineral that our bodies need for lots of functions. Deficiency is a known cause of migraines.

Magnesium occurs naturally in halibut (a fish), spinach & dark green leafy veggies, nuts, seeds and whole grains. White flour has very little magnesium left after processing. More information is at The National Institutes of Health Office of Dietary Supplements.

When you look at the Recommended Daily Allowance (RDA) remember that's a number that prevents sickness. It's not a number that promotes health. There is a difference.

In the case of a deficiency, it may take a while to build up a sufficient amount of magnesium (or other nutrients) again. It may take several months to notice results. And then one day you will realize that your headaches are fewer and less painful or gone.

Another cause of magnesium deficiency may be all the food additives, pesticides, herbicides and other products of chemistry labs that are added to highly-processed fake food.

Whenever you add a supplement to your diet, make a note and watch for changes.

3. Excessive computer usage. Children used to get lots of movement and exercise. Now we have children who use the computer or computer games a lot. They get little exercise so they don't use all of their muscles and this non-activity causes poor posture.

Headaches are caused by poor posture. Forward-head posture causes muscle strain in the neck and at the base of the skull.

Do you or your child have tight upper shoulders? They aren't supposed to be tight and hard.

4. Scoliosis, or curvature of the spine, is another cause of head pain. This is sometimes seen after hormone changes that come with puberty occur. Sometimes scoliosis is caused by asymmetries in anatomy but it can also be caused by habitual postures such as always leaning to one side while watching television.

5. Dietary sensitivities can also cause migraines, but again, this is not something that USED to cause migraines as much because we used to eat more real food.

6. Carrying heavy backpacks or shoulder bags also causes strained neck muscles. A rolling bag is better.

7. Playing musical instruments often causes forward-head posture which also causes muscle strain and head pain.

What can you do?

1. Do everything you can to fix your child's diet (and your own.) Get rid of the most likely food triggers (i.e., aspartame, peanuts.) Eat healthy, and if possible, eat organic. If you would spend 50 cents or a dollar on a candy bar, why not for an apple?

2. Get your child and yourself a good multi-vitamin/mineral supplement. Ask a knowledgeable clerk at a health food store. Take it daily. If it makes you more comfortable, ask your doctor, too.

3. Talk to your doctor if you suspect your headache is an indication of something serious. Your doctor can determine if you have a magnesium deficiency. He or she can also determine whether you have a condition that requires immediate treatment.

4. Observe your or your child's posture. Make helpful corrections based on the new knowledge you will have from this book.

Now you know lots of potential reasons for head pain. It's important to make changes to prevent future head pain. There are many natural, effective therapies including dietary changes, supplementation with magnesium, exercising and having physical fun to use all of your muscles and possibly postural correction to get rid of your headaches.

Tight muscles in the upper back

Are headaches caused by tight muscles in your neck, upper back and shoulder blades?

They surely can be! Here is a question from a reader that may be exactly what you need to know:

Here is the question:

I've been suffering with awful headaches for years now. I have what I call "knots" in my neck, upper back, shoulder blade area, and shoulders.   I've been to many doctors, I'm in physical therapy right now, and nothing has helped. I'm looking for exercises that I can do to break up these "knots". The headaches are becoming unbearable. They start at the base of my skull and radiate through my head, into the front of my face. I can't wait to feel like myself again. Please help.

Here is my answer:

I do not think there is anything that interferes more with life than head pain. Here are my best long distance thoughts.

You may need a massage therapist to help you relax the muscles that are causing these headaches and knots in your muscles. I will also give you self-help ideas.

The reason you have the headaches could be because trigger points in your upper shoulders and neck are 'firing' pain into your head. Those muscles are 'tight' and develop trigger points because they are over-stretched. This happens because of shortened muscles in your chest or your mid back. The shortened muscles pull on your shoulder and back muscles and cause them to complain and develop trigger points and muscle knots.

But the REAL problem, the real cause, starts in the shortened muscles in the chest and side of your armpit, in a nutshell. Maybe the front of your neck, too. They are pulling you forward and causing the pain and tightness in your upper back.

So why did those front muscles get short?

Well, the problem is usually posture. If you are always bent forward or have forward-head posture the muscles in front get short. When they become used to being short they become tight. Then they can hold you in a forward-bent posture.

Because bodies are logical and work in specific ways I can almost bet that your head pain is related to your posture. If one thing happens, then something else will happen. It has to. The result is pain.

But that's okay. Why? Because this pain is muscle-related and muscles are treatable!

If you go to a massage therapist be sure to interview that person first. Here's how to interview a massage therapist and find one who will be able to help you:

http://simplepainrelief.com/2009/11/22/how-to-find-a-massage-therapist-who-can-relieve-your-pain/

Or you can just go to http://SimplePainRelief.com and go to the Categories on the right hand side. There you will find a Massage Category. Clicking that link will take you to several articles about how and why massage works and what to expect. If you scroll, scroll, scroll through the articles in the Massage Category you will find the article about how to interview a massage therapist.

http://simplepainrelief.com/category/massage/

Wait! Muscles cause head pain?

You bet your boots they do! Not all of the time, of course, because there can be other causes, too, but *most* of the time.

Muscles can cause head pain when they are strained, tight, short, weak or unhappy for any reason. They can also develop trigger points and we will go into detail about trigger points in the next chapter.

The good thing about muscles causing pain is that muscles can be treated naturally with massage or other manual therapies.

Unfortunately, most doctors are not trained to know that muscles cause pain. When you are done reading this book you will know more about this and about your body than most doctors know.

What are trigger points?

Trigger points (TrP's or TP's) are very irritable places in muscles that cause pain. There are several types of trigger points. Sometimes you are quite aware of them, sometimes not. It depends on the type of TrP. The good thing about them is they can be released or relaxed and stop causing pain.

And do you know why they are called trigger points? It's because they "fire" pain elsewhere. Sometimes the pain is where the trigger point is but often it's at a distance from the TrP and you would never have guessed to work there.

A TrP is NOT: A knot or a ropey place in a muscle, a muscle spasm or contraction. The therapist cannot feel a TrP. They might feel the knot or tight area in muscle or soft tissue and it might have a TrP in it but there is no way to know if that is a TrP unless you say, "Yes, that causes my pain!" Or sometimes you might say, "When you press there my pain becomes less."

YOU can feel the TrP because you will feel it cause or refer pain elsewhere.

How do you treat a trigger point?

Sometimes you can pick up or lift the muscle that has the TrP. Other times you just press into it. Hold the pressure on the TrP for about 12 seconds then release the muscle. You can go back to the same TrP several times.

When you feel as though you or your therapist isn't pressing as hard anymore that's good! It means the muscle is relaxing. The TrP is relaxing. That's the goal.

An example of a trigger point

Here's an example of how a TrP can act:

I was working with a client who had head pain. When I picked up the muscle in her neck called SCM and applied some pressure to it she said, "You are holding my headache right between your fingers!"

The pain was in her HEAD but a trigger point in her NECK muscle (the SCM) was the cause of the pain. I could have rubbed the painful area of her head until the cows came home and it would not have helped her at all.

But by understanding TrP's I knew there was a good chance her headache was being caused by a TrP in her neck.

All bodies tend to follow the same pain patterns. There are charts that show you where pain typically is AND where the pain comes from. They show you the TrP that is causing the pain. Naturally, they are called trigger point charts.

Trigger points which cause head pain

Following are pictures of some common trigger points and the pain they cause. Areas of brighter red or denser dots indicate areas where painful or uncomfortable sensations are happening. The more red or density you see, typically the more pain.

Everyone's pain is not exactly in the same places so your pain may be in the same areas or slightly different. The location of the TrP's can also vary a bit from person to person but they do tend to be in muscles that are over-used or over-stretched.

The X's mark the spots where you would apply pressure. The X's are the locations of the TrP's.

There are lots of other trigger points but these are some of the most common head pain producers. And they are muscles that you can learn to treat yourself.

Occipital Muscles

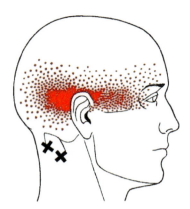

This picture shows the head pain that can be caused by the occipital muscles on either side of the back of your neck. These muscles attach from your neck bones to the base of your skull. Do you see the X's? Those are the TrP's to press, right at the bottom edge of the skull. You can also press onto the bone. When those muscles soften you can press even deeper, slightly underneath the skull. They will be tender and you may be able to tell that they are the cause of your head pain when they are pressed. Cold packs also work well to help these muscles relax.

A headache that feels like your whole head is being squashed can start with these muscles.

There are other muscles in the same approximate area that cause a variety of head pain. If you find any areas back there which are tight or refer pain elsewhere, treat them with pressure, too.

Temporalis Muscles

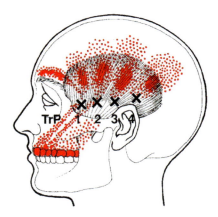

This picture shows how head pain can be caused by temporalis muscle TrP's. The temporalis muscle is grey and oval in this picture. You have one on each side of your head. It is a chewing muscle. If you place the palms of your hands on the sides of your head and pretend to chew you will feel the temporalis moving.

The temporalis muscles can cause pain over a large area and even into the teeth. There are stories of people having teeth removed because they thought the teeth were decayed. After extraction they still had 'tooth pain' because that wasn't the problem in the first place.

The four TP's (TrP's) are in the lower part of the temple muscles. You might not have all four; a whole muscle doesn't have to be involved; sometimes only part of the muscle has TP's.

Press or push UP into the muscle rather than pressing IN. You can also help the temporalis relax by weaving your fingers through your hair close to your scalp and clenching your fingers.

When you close your fingers you should feel your hair pulling on your scalp. Hold the pull for several seconds or until your fingers get tired. This is a good pull to use all around your head. It's called Cranial Fascial Release. That means head-fascia soft tissue release. Fascia is a type of soft tissue and soft tissue is everything that isn't bone.

Upper Trapezius Muscles

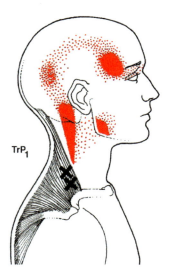

This picture shows the pain pattern caused by the upper trapezius muscles. There is one on each side of your body as with all of the pictures you will see here. The lined area is the muscle. It attaches to your collar bone, as you see in this picture.

This is the muscle that prefers to be unrolled from front to back rather than pressed into from the back or top.

The TrP's can be accessed by pressing in from the front. The farther out toward your shoulder you start feeling the sooner you will run into the upper 'trap'. It feels like a ridge or roll of firm muscle. Press into it from the front. Try to roll it toward your back. Tender? That means it needs a little treatment or love. Or, maybe a lot.

Once when I referred to the 'upper trap' a client asked me, "Is it called the trap because everything gets trapped there?" It's not but I said that was good! Muscle tension really does seem to get trapped there.

And why do we get muscle tension in the upper traps? Forward head posture and rounded shoulders are primary causes along with seats that lean back too far; things like that.

SCM Muscles

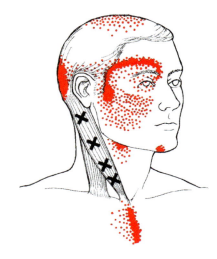

The muscle you are looking at here is the SCM or sternocleidomastoid. Wow! Look at all the areas of pain that little sweetie causes when it has TrP's!

That long name comes from the places it attaches to: The sternum (breastbone), the collarbone and the mastoid area of the skull behind the ear. This muscle has two sections. In the drawing you see the TrP's in the front section along with all the areas of pain they can cause. There is another section of this muscle and you will see that in the next picture.

Look in the mirror. Clench your jaw muscles. Do you see the two muscles on your neck that pop out when you clench? They form a V from the notch in your collar bone to behind your ears. Those are your SCM's.

These muscles can actually be lifted or picked up and rolled between your fingers like a piece of rope or garden hose.

Turn your head slightly toward the side that you want to treat and tilt your head slightly toward your chest. That softens the SCM and makes it easier to lift. And this is one you want to lift because you don't want to be pushing fingers into your throat.

It's easier to work cross body with this muscle. So if you are treating the left side, use your right hand.

When you have the muscle between your thumb and fingers, pick it up a bit and roll it back and forth. Treat the whole length of the SCM from collarbone to skull. Fibers of the muscle attach to your breastbone down for a few inches and also up onto your skull for a few inches so be sure to apply pressure to those boney areas, too.

If you have a lot of headaches with pain in the areas that this picture shows, your SCM may feel very tight to you. It may feel more rigid and less soft and flexible. If so, that means it's really tight and needs extra attention.

This pain pattern for SCM, as well as the pain pattern for upper trap, is very similar to the pain pattern of one-sided migraine headaches. For this reason, patients are often diagnosed as having migraines when their head pain actually comes from TrP's in the SCM.

TrP's in the SCM can be released and the head pain goes away.

But migraines are different. TrP therapy may help momentarily with migraine pain but the migraine will not go fully away or will come right back shortly after pressure is released.

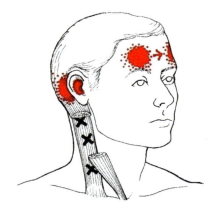

This picture shows the other leg of the SCM. The front part of the muscle has been cut away for the drawing. This part of the SCM is kind of tucked behind the front part. Sometimes you will be picking up both parts of the SCM without realizing it. That's fine.

Do you see the forehead pain? You could rub there forever and it wouldn't help because the cause of the pain is in your neck.

The TrP's are treated in the same way as the front part of the SCM.

Massater Muscles

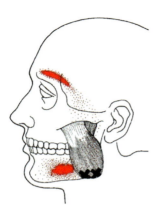

In this picture you are looking at the strong, strap-like jaw muscle that helps you chew. It's called the massater. The areas of pain are in the brow and side of the lower jaw with a lesser amount of discomfort connecting the two areas. The TrP's are at the most lower portion of the muscle.

You get to them by placing one clean finger way down at the bottom of your cheek on the inside of your mouth and pressing slightly down and out. Do this while supporting your muscle from the outside with your other hand.

If you are treating the left massater you would use the index or middle finger of your right hand side to apply pressure inside your left cheek. And you would support the muscle on the outside of the cheek with your left hand.

Assess your headache posture

1. Lie on your back. Do this on the floor if you can. Are the backs of your shoulders touching the floor? That's good. But if they are not touching the floor that means the muscles in the front of your shoulder are short.

Here's something that can help: Try to press your shoulders to the floor. This movement helps strengthen the muscles in your upper back and it ALSO stretches and lengthens the short chest muscles.

Do it only a few times so you don't get soreness from over-exercising those muscles. They will get stronger and you can do more and more of these shoulder presses over time. Just start gradually, please.

2. Look in the mirror. Is your right shoulder lower than the left? If so, that means the muscles next to your armpit in back and front and along that side of your back are probably short. The muscles on that side of your waist may also be shortened and tight. They need to be lengthened.

Side stretches will help. Stretch the shorter or lower side 4 times as much as the other side. Stretching the lower side 4 times as much is what allows change and muscular balance from side to side.

3. When you catch yourself in a mirror or window do you notice your head leading the rest of you? Is it out in front of your body? That's forward-head posture. It can also indicate that you have flat feet and would benefit from arch supports in your shoes.

4. Do you slouch and slump and sit on your tail bone? That causes forward-head posture as well as other postural dysfunction and pain.

5. Are the tops of your shoulders tight and hard? They are probably straining to hold up your heavy forward head.

6. Does your lower back hurt? That's a clue, too.

How does posture cause head pain?

I'll bet your doctor doesn't look at your posture when you tell him or her about your head pain. Most don't. But, she should!

Poor posture is the most common cause of headaches.

Why? Poor posture makes muscles unhappy and screaming muscles are responsible for most of our pain.

Tight muscles pull on bones. Tight muscles cause bone spurs (arthritis.) Tight muscles press on nerves and blood vessels. Overstretched muscles develop trigger points which "fire" pain into other parts of your body, sometimes quite far away. Weak muscles can't hold you up.

Muscles rule!

To be fair, there are a few doctors who do look at posture. When they don't, it's because they haven't been trained in physical medicine or because they simply don't have time.

I know you are getting the idea now: Poor posture is responsible for almost all pain and dysfunction, including headaches.

When your posture fails, it puts a lot of strain on your muscles. Your muscles become unhappy and cause symptoms like head pain.

Can you correct your posture?

It took a while for you to get into poor posture and it'll take a while for your body to remember how to be tall again. But, you can do it!

The muscles in the front of your body have shortened. Maybe your shoulders are rolled forward. Those muscles need to be relaxed or lengthened. Massaging and stretching these short muscles will help.

The muscles in your back—and the whole backside of your body except your calves—need to be strengthened.

In a nutshell, here are two keys for fixing your posture:

1. Lengthen the muscles in the front of your body.

2. Strengthen the muscles in the back of your body.

When you start correcting your posture you will be on the road to getting rid of your headaches. We will talk about this more.

How to tell if your posture is good or poor

Is your posture good or not-so-good?

People with poor posture look like they are leaning or collapsing forward. Often their head is way forward in front of their body ("forward head posture.") The curve in their neck is either too much or too flat, and so is the curve behind their waist. Their shoulders round forward.

Poor posture impacts a LOT of your body! Almost every part of your body is affected by collapsed posture. It even causes disorders of old age because it squashes your organs.

Here are several things to check so you will know whether your posture is good or not-so-good.

1. Stand up and hold your arms at your sides in their usual position. Look down. If your thumbs are pointing to each other that means your shoulders are rounded forward. Your chest muscles are tight and shortened and are pulling your shoulders forward. But, if your thumbs point straight ahead, your shoulders aren't rounded forward.

2. Are you constantly straightening up and constantly collapsing forward again? That's a clue that the muscles in the front of your body are short and pulling you into forward-head posture. It's also a clue that your back muscles are weak.

3. Are your feet flat or do you have nice arches? Flat feet will cause your posture to collapse because flat arches move your weight forward onto your toes. When that happens you lose muscle balance and you will develop a forward head posture.

4. Does the front of your neckline choke you or always slide backward? This can absolutely be related to #3.

5. Do you get a lot of headaches or pain in your neck or back? Those are symptoms caused by poor posture. They are also clues that your posture may be not-so-good.

And, I have good news for you!

When your posture is better you will have less pain in your head, back, arms...all over! And you will look better, too.

Remember, lengthen the front muscles and strengthen the back muscles.

Are you sure posture causes head pain?

Oh Boy! It surely can! In fact, it does.

Poor or collapsed posture can cause pain in your head, neck, feet, legs, hips, upper back and lower back. Why? Because being out of muscular balance means that you are using muscles to do the job of bones. Those poor muscles are weak, strained or stretched too far and they are not happy!

When a muscle is overworked or overstretched because it's trying to support you, it goes into contraction. There are two types of common contractions: (1) plain old short muscle contraction (a concentric contraction) and (2) the contractions that happen in weak muscles that are overstretched (an eccentric contraction.)

The muscles that are in contraction from being overstretched (like upper back and neck muscles) are the ones that complain loudest.

Poor posture can even cause your organs—heart, lungs, intestines, stomach—to have difficulty functioning. Why? Because you are collapsing forward and your heart, your lungs, your intestines and all of your organs are getting compressed or squashed. It is much harder for your organs to do their best job when they are squashed.

Steps to correct your posture

Here's an easy and quick way to strengthen the muscles in your upper back and the back of your neck. Wait–why do you need to strengthen those muscles?

Here's why:

1. A weak back hurts and causes head pain. A strong back holds you upright and avoids head pain.

2. When the muscles in the front of your neck and upper body are stronger (and shorter) than the back neck muscles your head goes forward. A 'forward head' causes upper back pain and muscle strain.

Okay. Here's an easy way to start to strengthen your back and neck muscles:

This is SO easy–you can do it in bed. When you are lying flat on your back you are in pretty neutral posture; your head is about where it should be and you don't have to think about your posture.

It's easier to get strong muscles in your back and neck when gravity isn't pulling you forward as it likes to when you are standing or sitting.

If you need a small neck roll to support your neck in a natural curve, that's fine.

Or, if you need a small flat pillow or folded hand towel behind your head to avoid neck strain, that's fine, too. Maybe at a later date you will discover that you don't need to prop your head as much. That's the goal.

1. Squeeze your shoulder blades toward your spine. Hold for several seconds. If you can't do it then just pretend you are doing it. Your body will start to remember after a while. This helps strengthen the muscles in your upper back.

2. Position your head in the most comfortable position, as close to neutral as possible. Gently press your neck into the mattress. GENTLY! Hold for several seconds. This activates the muscles in the back of your neck and strengthens them.

Always do these movements thoughtfully, slowly and gently. This isn't a race. Strength will come over time.

NOTE: Always start slowly! Do just a couple of times the first and second days. Then you can add one or two more movements each day.

If you do too many too soon you will have soreness just because the muscles are doing something they haven't done in a while. You might even get a headache so go slowly and thoughtfully. Pay attention to what you are feeling.

Do you have flat arches?

You may be able to tell from your wet footprint on a sidewalk. Does it show an arch? Hopefully, it shows both arches. Or does your footprint look flat?

Here's another way:

Stand up with your weight the same on both feet for 5 minutes. Then assess: Do you feel that most of the pressure on your feet is in your toes?

Feet are supposed to have arches. They are the foundation of your whole skeleton. Ideally, your weight should be pretty evenly distributed on your heels, the outsides of your feet and the balls and toes of your feet.

Just like a building, you need a solid foundation. If your foundation flattens, or collapses, the integrity of your building–your body–is compromised. We get into trouble, and the trouble starts with poor or collapsed posture.

If you need arch supports get a pair with a "real" arch, something that will truly support you. A running shoe store can be a good place to get arch supports.

Some arch supports may feel as though you have a **boulder** under your foot. That can be because your feet aren't used to them.

Try to get a pair that actually fits to the shape or your foot. If you have a long arch, you need a support that also has a long arch. You want the supports to hold your feet into the arched position they used to have.

Take time to adjust to the arch supports. Start with just an hour a day, then 2 hours. Work your way up to wearing them all day.

Here's something that will help your feet adjust:

Massage your feet by pressing the sole of your feet against a tennis ball or golf ball and rolling it back and forth, width-wise and length-wise. Do this with as much pressure as possible without too much discomfort. Standing is ideal. Support yourself with one foot while you roll the other foot. Do this for 5 minutes for each foot. If you need to hold onto something for balance, please do.

After you massage the first foot you will have one happy foot. You'll have to do your other foot so it will be happy, too. This helps relax your muscles and tendons in your feet and legs and make it easier to adjust to your new arch supports.

There is more to do to correct your posture and get you back to feeling and functioning well, but arch supports are a good place to start if your feet are flat.

Are migraines different?

Your head may actually pound. Light hurts your eyes. Every tiny sound is noise and the noise is all too loud. You might even throw up. You feel bad, and you look bad, too.

I really can't think of anything worse than a really bad migraine. A broken leg may keep you from moving but a migraine headache keeps you from **being**!

Migraines come in variations. Some are worse than others and some are horrible. They affect every system in your body.

Some people believe that headaches and migraines are closely related. I'm one of those people. For years and years, I never had "just a headache." Each time I started with a headache, I ended up with a migraine.

The best ways to avoid migraines are to have perfect posture and to avoid anything that can trigger your head pain. For those of us who are prone to headaches and migraines, any little strain on the muscles around our neck or head can and will cause pain.

Keeping a strong back, including the muscles in the back of your neck, helps a huge amount because it keeps you from getting strained neck muscles.

Recap: Good posture will make a big difference in the frequency and severity of your head pain. It's important to have good posture when you sit or stand.

You also need to prop your neck and head correctly when you sleep. More about that later.

What is a migraine headache?

Migraines are a type of severe head pain. They are called vascular headaches which means blood vessels are contracting and expanding. Why does this happen? It could be from your body chemistry, food sensitivities or irritated nerves that send messages to the blood vessels.

How do the nerves get irritated? Again, it could be body chemistry or food sensitivities and it could be from sitting, sleeping, working or moving in a way that causes bones or muscles to press on the nerves.

Nerves hate pressure!

What helps a migraine RIGHT NOW?

 Avoiding a migraine in the first place is a much better strategy than trying to get rid of it after you are already hurting.

But, when a migraine sneaks up or flat out attacks despite your best efforts here are a few tips to help ward off or lessen your pain.

1. Ice the base of your skull. Use a cold pack and put yourself in the most comfortable position you can. Use a thin towel or napkin between your skin and the cold pack. You can ice up to 20 minutes and then take a break so you don't injure your tissue. I just move the cold pack to a slightly different location.

Ice is typically the best treatment for nervy pain. There are lots of nerves in necks so the chances of your nerves being involved are good. Cold therapy also works well for muscles in most folks so that makes cold a good choice for a bad headache. You can use cold packs on your neck and do the next tip at the same time.

Interestingly, I have been outside in freezing cold winter weather shivering like crazy and had migraine headaches disappear before the car warmed up. I haven't figured out how to duplicate that in the summer.

2. Place a cold, almost dripping wet, cloth on your forehead and eyes. You can flip it over as it warms up from your heat. You can keep a pan of ice water next to the bed to re-wet and re-chill the cloth. You can put a plastic bag under a towel behind your head. That will keep your bed dry. The cold drips running down your face act to distract you and to numb nerves.

3. Compress your skull by wrapping your head in a long towel so that it is like a turban. Cover your eyes and ears with the turban, too. Make it as comfortably tight as you can. The idea is to compress your head and squeeze it (but don't squash your eyes.) This is comforting, blocks out noise and light, and helps reduce the pain of a migraine headache.

4. If you can take the time to lie down, warming your feet and hands can help. Chill your head and neck and warm your hands and feet with extra covers or hot water bottles.

5. Aspirin may not touch a migraine, but two tablets of Alka Seltzer taken at the very beginning of a migraine attack often knocks out the migraine. I suspect this happens because it releases the whole dose of aspirin all at once rather than gradually. Try this only if you aren't allergic to aspirin. It may be a way to avoid taking more heavy-duty headache medicine.

What else gets rid of head pain?

Here are some other simple head pain relief tips and remedies to try:

1. If the muscles on the tops of your shoulders are all "jammed up," try a heating pad or heated cloth bag filled with rice to relax your shoulders. If you apply heat to your neck your head may feel worse. If that happens, you will know that cold therapy is the better choice.

2. Hike your shoulders to your ears and hold them there for several seconds. Squeeze them up, up, up. Now relax. Do this a few times while being sure to hold your head on top of your shoulders rather than letting it be in front of your body. This movement will help fatigue the shoulder muscles so they won't be so tight. This is a good one to do when you don't have a headache, too.

3. Push gently, stretch and pull on the muscles around your ears, temples, forehead, back of your head or anywhere you can reach. Explore and see what's tight or tender. Sometimes a migraine comes from the inside out and sometimes from the outside in. The pain patterns look much the same. It's easier to treat the migraines that are really coming from the muscles on the outside. That's because they are caused by trigger points rather than nerves and blood vessels inside the head and neck.

4. Pull your hair. The soft tissues around your whole head get tight with a migraine or tension headache. By clasping your fingers in your hair, close to your head, you can use your hair as little levers to help relax your scalp muscles. Clasp close to your skull and you will feel the hair pulling when you close your fingers. Work your way around as much of your head as you can. Take your time. If your hands get tired, rest.

5. Try to straighten up. If you can lift your breastbone, your head will move back and be more over your body and take some of the strain off your muscles and nerves.

Do this when you DON'T have a headache or migraine, too. Many people can tell instantly that lifting the breastbone and squeezing the shoulder blades together gives relief.

6. If you sleep several hours in a row and wake with head pain try this: Do something to wake yourself sooner, every two or three hours, so you can change position even if it's only briefly. Set an alarm or drink a large glass of water before bed and every time you wake up. Your bladder can act as an alarm clock when it gets full.

Will doing that interfere with your sleep? Yes. But if it prevents head pain you may decide it's worth it.

Does exercise help head pain?

1. Years ago, I remember reading an article in a health magazine that said some people are able to actually exercise their migraines away. Some people do aerobic exercise, like fast walking or running or jogging in place, and their migraine headaches go away.

I mean, come on. Can you imagine jogging when your head hurts just being still?

More recently, I read a medical article about migraines and a researcher-doctor said he also gets migraine relief when he does aerobic exercise. So it might be worth a try.

2. Here's another thing about exercise and migraines and being out of balance. If you have some upper body and neck muscles that are weak and others that are too tight ("out of balance") they don't support your head where it should be. That allows muscle strain and trigger points to develop.

By starting an exercise program which is designed to get your head back over your shoulders where it belongs you can begin to get rid of your headaches.

This ideal exercise program would strengthen all of the muscles of the back of your body except for your calves. Calves are supposed to be soft.

All of the muscles from your knees to the back of your neck are probably weak and need to become stronger. When they are stronger they will help hold your heavy head over your shoulders. And, that's where your head belongs: Over your shoulders not in front of them.

As an added bonus, not only will you have fewer headaches you will feel better all over

PLEASE NOTE: Whenever you do movements for your neck always do them carefully, slowly and thoughtfully. Pay close attention to what's going on so you don't aggravate your touchy neck and cause a headache.

Does Yoga help head pain?

How can yoga help relieve your headaches? Oh, let me count the ways:

It relaxes the muscles around your chest, ribs, shoulders and neck. These are the same muscles that get tight and cause headache symptoms.

Yoga helps reduce your stress. When you're feeling all stressed your muscles clamp down on nerves that go to your head.

It helps strengthen the muscles of your backside, and makes you long and strong; it creates muscular balance. A strong back and a long, strong body helps you have good posture. Good posture, with your head over your body instead of out in front, reduces headaches.

Yoga gets your circulation moving and that helps move the metabolic (body) wastes out of your body. It reduces swelling which can also be a cause for head pain.

It helps you become more "in tune" with your body. When your muscles start to complain or your head starts to hurt you will be able to figure out the cause and correct it.

Yoga can help reduce your blood pressure but if you are having headaches from high blood pressure you'd better get to a doctor immediately!

So, yoga is a full-body stretching and strengthening movement program with a LOT of benefits.

If you take a class, always remember: It's your body. If a move doesn't feel appropriate to you or feels like it will make your head hurt or your headache feel worse DON'T DO IT. Instead, practice a different movement (pose) or breathing.

Yoga helps take the pressure off the muscles around your head and neck by correcting your posture. It helps short muscles lengthen and weak muscles get stronger. It promotes muscle balance. Yoga helps improve your breathing.   That's good since shallow breathing could also be a cause of your headaches by not giving you enough oxygen.

That's how yoga can help you get rid of your headaches.

Do legs cause head pain?

Migraines can be caused by having a short leg.

According to a study by the US Army, approximately one out of ten people have an actual leg length difference. Additionally, about one out of one hundred people have pelvic bones which are smaller on one side than the other side.

According to myofascial (muscle and soft tissue) pain experts Drs. Travell and Simons a leg length difference of 1/8 inch or more puts you at risk for pain and dysfunction. Why? Because your body does things like tilt, twist or rotate automatically to try to correct or adapt or accommodate that difference.

There are two types of "short legs." Both can cause migraines or headaches.

1. One is an actual anatomical difference which could be caused by severe injury or polio or nature and is measurable on x-rays. It could be either the upper or the lower leg bones.

2. The other type is a functional leg length difference. That means the bones are all the same length but muscles in the body cause one hip to hike or tilt so your body acts like one leg is shorter but it's really not. Your hips can move independently of each other so it is possible to have one hip that is higher or more forward than the other. There is a muscle on either side of the waist called the QL that can cause functional leg length difference. When it gets tight it will pull on the hip bones on the short side and hike the leg.

People with a leg length difference often have migraines because walking with a tilt puts a lot of strain on the muscles at the base of the skull. It causes a rotation (slight turning) of the head. That can affect the nerves and blood vessels which play a part in migraines. Those people can have other pain, too, such as hip pain on one side or low back pain or TMJ (jaw joint) dysfunction.

Can you fix leg length differences?

Good news! There is a relatively easy fix so you don't have to go through life out of balance and with migraines.

ANATOMICAL SHORT LEG: Lifting your entire foot on the short leg side enough to level your hips will go a long way in helping you feel better, have fewer migraines, and fewer problems with your neck and muscles.

This requires that you only wear certain shoes. They must have a solid, thick hard rubber sole. A shoemaker can split a firm rubber sole and add a layer of neoprene rubber to lift the short leg. This doesn't work with air or gel type shoes. A shoe can also be built up by adding more material to the bottom of the sole.

Also, if you have a really skilled shoemaker or cobbler he might be able to remove your whole sole and replace it with a new, thicker sole. High heels can be built up, too. Talk to your shoe repair man.

It may seem like a lot of work or you might not want to give up your stylish shoes but the benefits to your body are huge.

FUNCTIONAL SHORT LEG: A skilled massage therapist can help relax and release the tight out-of-balance muscles that are pulling your bones out of neutral. Many Chiropractors also claim to be able to re-align the hip bones. Tight muscles will move the bones back out of position, though.

Clues to leg length differences

Perhaps one pant leg is always longer than the other. That was the clue for my 91 year old client who had back pain and migraines for over 70 years. His doctors never looked for or told him he had a leg length difference.

After we discovered it he told me, "My tailor always told me I did!" His anatomical leg length difference was about 2 inches. He had his shoe lifted in three stages so his joints and muscles could adapt gradually.

Do you remember the actor John Wayne? When I watched one of his old movies I realized that every time he stopped moving he stood in a particular way. He always put one leg out to the side and it was always the same leg. Why did he do this? It was his natural way of leveling his hips and eyes so he could function. John Wayne had a considerable difference in the lengths of his legs.

Maybe when you look in the mirror you can see that one shoulder is higher than the other or that your head sits off to the side instead of dead in the middle of your body. That's a clue, too.

Or, as you look in the mirror, does your belt line drop to one side?

Are you wearing blue jeans? Can you see more of one pocket than the other?

Those are clues that you may have a leg length difference.

How do you know how much lift you need?

A physical medicine doctor can take x-rays of your legs and hips when you are lying down and measure for you. Or, you can guesstimate by placing notebooks or magazines under your short leg and adding or removing pages until you feel more level and look more level in the mirror. Many neuromuscular and neurosomatic massage therapists are trained in measuring leg length differences.

When you have a pretty close measurement you can go to a shoemaker.

When you correct an anatomical or functional leg length difference it will stop the tilting and twisting that your body does automatically to try to level itself.   Then you can have fewer headaches and less body pain.

What is a tension headache?

Most headaches are caused by muscle tension. Tension headaches should more accurately be called Muscle Tension Headaches. Muscles are the most common cause of head pain. Almost always, in fact!

When your jaw gets tight or your head moves forward the muscles around your upper back, neck and face get strained and tight. Tight muscles clamp down on nerves and blood vessels. The result is a muscle tension headache.

Migraine headaches often start out as tension headaches for migraine sufferers.

What causes muscle tension?

Here are the most likely causes of discomfort that feel like pressure or squeezing at the base of your skull.

1. You slept with your neck 'too straight.' This happens when your pillow doesn't support your neck. It's more as though your neck is in a 'hammock' position. This strains the muscles at the base of your skull. Or you slept on your side without proper support for your head and neck.

2. You stick your chin out when you are trying to see the monitor or something else. This happens especially to people who wear bifocals because they are trying to read through the bottom of the lens and the screen is too high. This shortens the muscles at the base of your skull.

3. Sitting in a new or unusual position, perhaps with your head turned to the side.

4. Sleeping in a strange position with your head tilted.

5. Using a different chair or car or bed pillow.

6. Your regular chair or pillow.

7. Any prolonged position can cause muscle strain and tension in the muscles around your head, shoulders and neck.

8. Driving. Most car seats tilt back too far or have headrests that push your head forward. Either of these will strain the muscles that cause tension headaches.

9. Couches (sofas) and chairs that have too much backward lean and force you to move your head forward.

10. Slouching or sitting on your tailbone with a rounded back. Slouching or leaning sideways will do it, too.

11. Forward head posture or holding your head in front of your body.

If you take action, you can start to be rid of your headaches

Steps to get rid of tension headaches

Here are some solutions. You may need to try and use several.

1. Watch your posture. Try to keep it neutral and straight. A strong back will help with this.

2. Use a pillow or rolled towel behind your waist to help you sit upright.

3. Ice the back of your neck. Try to wrap your cold pack all the way down to the notch between your collar bones. Some people find heat to be more beneficial.

4. Pad the back of your car seat so you can sit more upright or farther away from the headrest if it's the kind that pushes your head forward.

5. Get a strong back including the muscles in the back of your neck and improving your posture.

6. Lift your chest so your head can move back more over your body where it is supposed to be.

7. Massage works. Either find a professional massage therapist or do it yourself. The back of your skull is called the occiput. Make sure the therapist knows how to massage there before you spend your money.

Basically, to do it yourself, press into the muscles at the base of your skull and in your upper neck and back. Use your thumbs or fingers. You will know when you are on a tender place! It will be tender because the muscles are tight and hurt when you press.

Those tender areas are the places to press on. Pressing will help them relax. You have to relax or release your upper shoulders, too.

8. Watch your posture and positions very carefully to avoid causing muscle strain. You may have to make changes in the way you sit, sleep and walk.

For years I had a love-hate relationship with walking.

I enjoyed the freedom, fresh air and seeing nature but hated the migraine that would almost always follow a nice walk. Finally I realized that I was turning my head way to the side to look at interesting things as I passed. That was straining my neck muscles.

I started rotating my whole upper body to the side instead of just my head. Kind of like I was swaying in the breeze. That saved my neck muscles and ended the headaches.

And, as you know, sometimes the muscles at the base of your skull are NOT the cause of your muscle tension headaches. Sometimes it's the muscles that stretch from the notch of your collar bones to behind your ears--the SCM's. You saw the trigger point pictures of them earlier.

Surgery for headaches?

A recent research article stated that a specific type of surgery could get rid of migraines and cluster headaches.

The surgery involved cutting muscles at the base of the patient's skull. When these muscles were cut, pressure from the muscles that caused the headache was released.

Without pressure from the muscles, the head pain could go away.

But, surgery is invasive.

It causes injury to the tissues.

It causes scars.

It is expensive.

And, surgery can have side effects and after-effects that are not desired.

The researchers had already figured out that the headaches were caused by muscles. They knew that the symptom (the head pain) was caused by tightness in the muscles under the base (back) of the skull.

But, they did not look at therapies which were less invasive and already available.

The reason they didn't may be because the researchers simply did not know there are natural, simple and effective muscular therapy techniques that relieve pain. Or it might be because there is much more money to be made from surgical procedures. (Oops! Did I say that?)

Fact #1: The roles of muscles and other soft tissues as causes of pain are largely overlooked in the medical field. This is not widely taught in medical schools.

Fact #2: Methods of treating or releasing muscles are also not well known in conventional medicine. Again, this is barely "touched" on in medical schools.

Fact #3: Tight muscles can be released manually. That means pressure from fingers, hands, forearms, elbows or tools like tennis balls can release the muscles and eliminate your pain.

The muscles we are talking about here are called occipital muscles. They are located under the occipital bone which is the lowest part of the back of your skull. You saw the trigger point picture for them earlier.

Since muscles tend to work together as a group many of your muscles may be tight in this area.

And, as you know, tight muscles can entrap (trap) nerves. They can also develop trigger points which cause pain. When do muscles often become tight? When they are overworked or over-stretched.

But muscles are not supposed to be hard and tight. They are supposed to be flexible and soft.

If your head is too far forward instead of over your body, where it belongs, you are overworking your occipitals. Also, if you wear bifocals and tilt your head back a lot, that will tighten your occipital muscles.

Painting a ceiling? That will do it, too.

Get rid of muscle tension headaches

Here are several ways to get rid of muscle tension headaches.

1. Go to a really good massage therapist who knows how to work deeply into the muscles at the back of your head and neck. She will warm all of the muscles in the area with her hands and then may use her fingers or a small rubber-tipped tool to press into these muscles. You may have to find a Neuromuscular or Neurosomatic Massage Therapist or Rolfer (these are massage specialties.)

2. You can 'dig' or press into these muscles yourself, but we usually can't do this as well as a massage professional. Still, you may have some good results with this. If it's tender, you know you are in the right place. Hold each spot for 12 seconds. You can go back to the most tender places several times, always for 12 seconds.

3, Try ice therapy. Use a bag of frozen peas or an ice pack that fits comfortably under your neck as you lie on your back. Place a pillow case or other thin fabric between you and the ice pack. Spend 20 minutes on and off. (Heat is generally best for releasing tight muscles and ice for nerves. But, since this area is so closely involved with irritated nerve fibers, ice usually seems to work best for softening occipital muscles.)

4. Scrunch up your shoulders to tire the muscles so they will relax.

Pressure on tight muscles will cause some discomfort. That's because they are actually tighter than they should be. But, when they are released, those muscles will no longer cause migraine or headache pain for you.

Headaches in the back of your head

Many muscles in your upper body can cause headaches in the back of your head.

1. Headaches in the back of your head can be caused by muscles in your upper shoulders (the trapezius muscles.) The trap muscles actually stretch way down toward your waist and the lower part of the traps, near the mid-point of your spine, can cause head pain, too.

2. Headaches can be caused by muscles in the back of your neck, at the base of your skull or even the muscles that run farther down along your spine.

3. Muscles in the *front* of your neck and skull can also cause headaches. You cannot treat the muscles in the front of your neck or at the base of your skull yourself but a Neuromuscular or Neurosomatic Massage Therapist with this specialized training can help.

If you treat as many of the muscles that you can reach yourself, but you still have a headache in the back of your head, it could be the anterior suboccipital or longus coli muscles.

4. And the SCM muscles which stem from the notch between your collar bones to the skull bone behind your ears can also cause pain in the back of your head.

What about massage for head pain?

Does massage help headaches? I truly believe in the value of massage therapy for getting rid of headaches quickly.

In fact, I believe in the value of massage period! It's old medicine and is all natural.

When the muscles in the upper back are massaged or treated they don't need to be treated gently. Thoughtfully and carefully yes but not gently. When muscles are tight and knotty they will feel tender. They may feel VERY tender. That's how you know you are in the right place when you search for trigger points.

If you just rub nicely it won't help. If you press, pinch or massage too deeply, it's too painful and the body won't respond as well. The pressure should be about a 6 or 7 on a scale of 1 to 10 with 10 being the most uncomfortable and 1 is nothing.

Some massage therapists don't get it; they just don't understand how bodies work. They might blast away on a suspected trigger point or knot or tight area for a whole hour and it won't relax. That's because it CANNOT relax. It is already over-stretched and doesn't want to be more stretched or relaxed.

All you get is sore and you will still have the knotted area.

If you suspect that's what's happening to you, educate your therapist. Tell him or her to work all AROUND that area and even on the opposite side of your body. If a tight area doesn't relax right away, that means something somewhere else is pulling on it and making the knot. The only way to get rid of the muscle tension in that case is to find and relax the muscles that are causing it.

Ask the therapist to work more deeply by unrolling the upper trapezius muscles. The trapezius muscles prefer being unrolled to being pressed.

Also ask her to treat the SCM (sternocleidomastoid) muscles by lifting them and rolling them between her fingers.

If massage hasn't worked for you, perhaps you need to find a therapist who understands trigger point work or who works with headaches. Every massage therapist has different training and some have excellent skills for helping you have natural relief for headaches.

Heat therapy or cold therapy?

The rule of thumb is cold for nervy pain and heat for muscles.

Use heat on the tops of your shoulders if they are tight, wrapping it around to your collar bones.

You can use either ice or heat at the base of your skull. If the heat makes you feel a little worse, that's a clue to use ice there.

I'd always go with cold therapy first on the neck because it has lots of muscles *and* lots of nerves.

Some people cannot use cold therapy due to medical conditions such as Reynaud's Syndrome.

Here's more info on using heat and cold therapy:

Go to http://SimplePainRelief.com. Scroll to the Categories on the right hand side. Go to the Category for Ice-Heat.

What's the best way to sleep?

Do most of your headaches occur during the night or as soon as you start to get out of bed? Then it's possible that sleeping positions and movements that strain your neck are responsible for your head pain.

It always amazes me that we can hurt ourselves even in our sleep, but we do.

Headaches don't happen without a reason. They happen because your neck, head or shoulder muscles get tight and cranky and complain. They let you know they are unhappy by creating head pain.

Pillows can help your head feel better or can make it feel worse.

Do you sleep on your side, your stomach or your back?

STOMACH SLEEPING:

Stomach sleeping puts a lot of strain on a neck and most stomach sleepers I know tell me they tend to sleep on the same side all the time. So, stomach sleeping isn't the best option for anyone. If you do that and can change it, your neck will thank you.

But, there is one benefit to stomach sleeping, especially if you could switch from side to side and not stay locked in one position. The benefit is it helps you maintain the slight curve in your low back that we are supposed to have. We need a slight low back curve in order to keep our head over our shoulders without neck muscle strain when we are upright. The curve goes in the direction of our abdomen or belly – forward, not rounded backward. The curve creates a slight hollow in the lower back.

BACK SLEEPING:

If you sleep on your back and your neck is pushed into a too-straight position during the night, either by your pillow or the lack of a pillow, that creates head pain. There are muscles on top of your shoulders, at the front/sides of your neck and at the base of your skull. If any of those get strained, a headache results. If you are prone to migraines, this is a good way to get one.

Also, if you sleep with a fat pillow pushing your head forward that can cause two problems.

1. It can definitely cause head pain.
2. It perpetuates the "head forward" posture that we would like to eliminate.

Here are three pillows which are helpful in maintaining the curve in the back of your neck and preventing waking up with a headache.

1. The Tempurdic pillow or a similar memory-foam type pillow. It softens and sinks under the weight of your head, but supports the backside of your neck. Warning: Most are *way too big* for back sleepers. Get a junior/child size or, at most, a medium size pillow.

2. Interestingly, a down "stomach sleeper" pillow is good for back sleepers. Fluff it up, punch to make a depression for your head, and enjoy. There should be enough down beneath your neck to keep a nice curve in it as you sleep. You can even pull up the wings, or bottom corners, of the pillow to stabilize your head. This is especially helpful if you get migraines during the night. It prevents you from tilting your head sideways and straining your neck muscles while sleeping.

3. You can make your own custom pillow from a fiberfill batt. This is similar to cotton batting, but it is made of polyester fiberfill, which is soft and cushy. You can buy a fiberfill batt (not the loose stuffing) at a fabric store or department.

Take it out of the package and roll it into a neck roll which feels like the correct size for your neck. If you feel you need a little more lift under your head, leave a tail on your roll. The flat tail will go under your head and the rounded neck roll goes under your neck.

You can simply place the part of the batt you are using into a pillow case and roll it up; no sewing necessary! You can always add more or take some away to be most comfortable. You can have two or three in different sizes around, and switch as desired. It's very inexpensive.

SIDE SLEEPING:

If you are a side sleeper and wake with a headache, the reason is most likely that your head and your neck was tilted either up or down. Your pillow is too fat or too flat. Your neck and base-of-skull muscles get shortened or pulled or strained during the night and those muscles cause your head pain or migraine.

Side sleepers should use a pillow which allows their spine and neck to be in neutral all night, not tipped chin to ceiling or floor. It's the tipping or tilting that causes neck and head pain. You may find it useful to stack two flatter pillows, or place a down pillow on top of a firmer pillow.

You can also generate your own custom pillow with fiberfill batts, as discussed above, and place it on top of your bottom pillow. You may find a nice, expensive pillow especially designed for side sleepers which has a firmer core and cushy outer layer.

The idea for side sleepers is to support your head in a neutral position AND to support your neck, also. That means slightly more cushioning under your neck.

The pillow has to be tall enough so that you don't mash your shoulder. Squashed shoulders cause head pain, too.

When you buy a pillow, check on the store's return policy. If you try it for a night or two and it doesn't work out for you, some stores will let you return it. That way you won't end up with a bunch of unusable pillows that cost a lot of money.

Some people say they just cannot change their sleeping habits or cannot fall asleep in a different position. These tips may help:

1. Practicing relaxation techniques while laying flat on the floor or bed may help your muscles get used to being in a different position.

2. Practicing deep breathing using your whole torso, chest and belly may allow you to slip into sleep in a new position.

3. Maybe a stretching or yoga class would be the ticket to wake up all of your muscles so they can relax in a different position.

What else causes morning head pain?

Sometimes you wake up feeling fine but by the time you get out of bed you have a headache or migraine. What's happening?

Here are some possibilities:

I would wake up feeling fine. No head pain. Then I would twist my neck and stretch my head around to see the alarm clock. That twist and stretch aggravated my neck enough that I would get an instant migraine!

It actually took me quite a long time to figure that out. It happened several times before I realized that I was causing those migraines with movements that aggravated nerves or blood vessels in my neck. When I quit doing that twist and stretch the morning head pain stopped.

Could that be your possibility? Or, perhaps you can think of something else you may be doing to cause your headache to start when you woke up feeling fine.

Does it feel like you're straining your neck by sitting straight up when you get out of bed? Try rolling onto your side and pushing yourself up with your arms while keeping your neck in a straight, neutral position.

One of my clients always awoke feeling fine, but by the time she was in the kitchen with her coffee, her head pain started. Right after she took the first deep drags on her cigarette, her headache started. Every morning.

What do you suppose was the cause of her headache?

Because she was a smoker, and because she inhaled strongly, using the muscles in her jaw and temples (the temple muscles work with the jaw muscles) she caused those muscles to become tight and restricted. That caused her morning headaches. Like many morning headaches once they started they tended to stay all day.

So the plan is to avoid your headache in the first place.

Pay attention to what may be creating head pain for you. Change the position, posture, activity or movement you suspect and see if that makes a difference.

A simple change could make all the difference in the world. Awareness is the first step in the right direction.

More about food and head pain

I had a friend who would get an instant migraine when she ate an orange. After a while, she started avoiding oranges. Other times, it is not an instant reaction. That's why keeping a food diary helps. You can see patterns after you eat certain things.

A varied and healthy diet with lots of fruits and vegetables helps for many reasons. One of the reasons is that constipation can create conditions for a migraine. It may be the pressure from the packed intestines on the blood vessels in the abdomen that causes a migraine, because migraines are vascular headaches. That means they are related to what is happening with blood vessels.

Keeping things moving through your intestines with a good diet helps prevent migraine. You might consider taking additional fiber from a bottle to avoid constipation. Also, many headache and other medicines cause constipation.

Monosodium glutamate (MSG) is a common head pain trigger. If you want to stay away from it, read labels. It's used in seasonings and flavorings and lots of processed foods.

When I suffered from seriously awful migraines I became aware of the cause and effect that food can have. After I eliminated the foods that triggered my migraines, the head pain became much less severe and much less frequent. Over the years since, I have continued to eliminate more "trigger" foods as I suspected them including chocolate, peanuts, pork and shellfish.

So, how do foods cause migraines and other pain?

Some foods can cause inflammation (irritation and swelling.) Inflammation in your tissues causes muscle aches and pains. Inflammation in your blood vessels can cause a migraine.

Food can also cause an allergic reaction. Some of us have serious allergic reactions which can put us in danger. When we discover such an allergy, for instance to peanuts, of course we stay away from peanuts.

We must also stay away from the foods that 'trigger' our headaches or migraines.

Sometimes we can identify a trigger food. If a food causes a symptom like a stuffy nose, or headache, or lots of mucus (causing throat clearing,) that's a clue. The reaction might occur very soon after eating something, but sometimes the head pain won't come for a while. That makes it harder to figure out.

You might have a lot of food triggers or you might only have some of the more common ones.

Sometimes it isn't actually the food--it is chemicals and other ingredients that are added to the food. MSG is a common additive which causes stuffy noses, migraines and headaches. Artificial sweeteners like aspartame also are common migraine triggers.

You might not realize that what you are eating is actually causing a large part of your head pain. It helps to keep a log and look for tie-ins.

Here are a few of the more common food triggers:

wine

aged cheese

pork

shellfish

citrus fruit

nuts, especially pistachios

peanuts

caffeine

chocolate and carob

There are lots more than this. And, not everyone gets a headache from the same foods. I've seen fruits on lists of migraine triggers that I ate frequently which never caused a migraine for me.

Sometimes you can get away with eating small amounts of a food, like nuts, as long as you don't do it too often. Sometimes, you won't be able to eat any at all.

There are things I haven't ingested in over 30 years because I didn't want to take the chance of a bad headache. Caffeine is one of those even though it is in many headache medications.

And I do still enjoy smelling chocolate. I just don't eat it.

You might remember the good old days when sugar was in your soda pop, gum, cereals and ice cream. Read the labels now, and chances are really good you will find high fructose corn syrup and artificial sweeteners, instead.

You have to read labels to find out what ingredients besides the ones you expected are being fed to you.

So, as you see, lots of times your head pain starts with what you put in your mouth.

Pain relief without drugs?

Is there any way to get rid of headaches and migraines naturally or are you doomed to take pain medication forever?

While pain medication or drugs like the triptans can definitely seem (and be) very useful in the treatment of migraines and other head pain, they do have a serious downside. All medicines have side effects and some are dangerous.

We see more ads for medicines than anything else because the big pharmaceutical (drug) companies can make a lot of money by "educating" us. It wouldn't make sense for them to educate us about natural products or methods of pain relief. There is not much profit in natural pain relief.

And, if we all got better they wouldn't make any money at all.

At any rate, drugs treat symptoms but they don't treat the reasons for head pain.

By now you have the knowledge to get rid of a lot of the causes of your head pain. If you take action, your headaches will become less severe and less frequent. If you do need to take medicine you will need less.

Are you a detective?

Symptoms, like headaches or back pain, happen for reasons. You won't get pain unless there is a cause.

The cause could be something that you ate, the way you sit or sleep, the way you hold the phone when you talk, drugs you take or the length of your leg bones. There are lots of triggers, reasons or causes for migraines and headaches.

Your job is to figure out what is causing your pain.

When you know what causes your symptoms, you can take action. If you don't take action, nothing will change. If you take control of your own health you can become pain-free or close to it.

Now, please don't get me wrong. I am grateful that we have options that sometimes include medicine or surgery. Sometimes a drug or surgical procedure is truly a life saver. But sometimes it has the opposite effect.

If you want to get rid of your headaches or migraines naturally, here are several questions to answer to get you started thinking about possible causes:

1. When does your headache start?

2. Does it wake you in the night? Could it be your pillow or your sleeping position?

3. Does your head pain come on 1/2 an hour after you get out of bed or after you get to work? What are you doing then? Do you smoke? Does it happen when you drive a specific distance?

4. Some foods or food additives cause headaches or migraines and they often come on within a short time after eating them. Have you noticed headaches after eating?

5. Where does your head hurt? The sides of your head? The back of your skull? Around your eyes?

6. Is your headache one-sided? Is it always the same side?

7. How is your posture when sitting, standing and sleeping?

8. Do you have a forward head? Are your upper shoulders tight?

9. Do you clench your jaw?

Answering these questions, and paying attention to where, when and how often your pain occurs will help you find the causes of your pain.

When you know the causes of your head pain, you can take steps to eliminate it naturally.

Improve your health & get rid of head pain?

Here are some of the ways you can improve your health and get rid of head pain at the same time:

1. Be responsible for your own wellness. No one cares as much about your body as you have to. Educate yourself about the causes of your pain.

2. Feed your body wholesome foods and avoid fake foods and additives. Just because it is sold in a grocery store does NOT mean the thing on the shelf is food! There is no fooling your body. When you eat junk your body knows!

3. Take a good multi-vitamin/mineral supplement. I do. I'm not a doctor but plenty of doctors take these to stay healthy, too. A magnesium deficiency can cause headaches and muscles function best when they have all of the nutrients that they need.

4. Reduce your stress. Take some time out for a stress-buster like meditation or yoga, tai chi or stretching.

5. Stretch in the correct directions. The correct direction is the one that you never or hardly ever use! Stretch in the OPPOSITE direction of the positions you use the most.

6. Breathe deeply. Move your ribs. Get the oxygen in.

7. Get enough sleep. People in research situations who are not allowed to sleep develop all-over muscle pain.

8. Drink sufficient water. Your muscles and cells need water to function and feel their best.

9. Become knowledgeable about your body and the causes of your pain. Educate yourself with trustworthy websites and books.

10. Take action. Do what you need to do to become pain-free, naturally. That's the only way you will get better and feel better. As the old saying goes, 'No one can do your pushups for you.'

11. Prop yourself carefully in bed so your head is supported and your neck spine is in line with your back spine.

12. Sit on your sit bones rather than on your tail bone.

So there you have it! You don't have to do them all at once but start at least one today. Just keep moving in the right direction and soon you really WILL be moving with less head pain and in better health, naturally!

Let's review

So, as you now know, migraines and headaches can have many causes including:

1. Sensitivities to certain foods or compounds or smells. Avoid them.

2. Hormone shifts. You may be stuck with them.

3. Posture. You can fix it.

4. A short leg or one flat foot. This is correctable.

5. Trigger points. These can be treated naturally.

Ha! I bet you didn't know about the last three before you read this book, did you? I'll bet your doctor doesn't, either. Most don't.

That's okay. My goal is to help you get rid of those miserable headaches.

Sometimes the only way to get better is to be your own doctor or therapist. Please don't get me wrong–I love doctors! Even surgeons! I wouldn't be here today talking with you otherwise.

But there is so much for them to know and so little time to spend with you. And mostly doctors learned about meds in med school. They didn't learn much about muscles or the causes of head pain. That's why you need to.

I have been where you are. Migraines used to take blocks of days out of my life but now if I sleep crooked and get a migraine it's much more controllable and rare.

In the end

I hope you have been able to discover some, many or all of the causes of your head pain. I'm counting on you to take action to feel better.

I put together a list of self-help books that can help you be your own doctor and therapist and help you get rid of your headaches and migraines naturally.

It's at http://budurl.com/migraine2   The list is at Amazon and it's a Listmania list. I have several lists but this one is for headache sufferers.

I wrote a paragraph for each book I recommend with more details about it. These books are all in my personal library because they are so valuable. You may be able to ask your local librarian to find them for you. If you have to buy just one, I'd go with the blue Trigger Point book by Clair Davies.

I'd also like to invite you to visit my natural self-help website http://SimpleBackPainRelief.com to learn more about getting rid of upper back muscle knots and pain.

You can find me and all of my self-help natural pain relief websites at http://KathrynMerrow.com

This book is the first in a series of natural pain relief books. You can find them at Amazon.com by typing in my name.

My goal is for you to get rid of your pain naturally!

Kathryn Merrow

Printed in Great Britain
by Amazon.co.uk, Ltd.,
Marston Gate.